TOP 30 SUPERFOODS
TO NATURALLY LOWER HIGH BLOOD PRESSURE

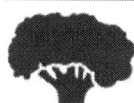 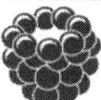 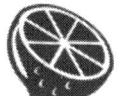 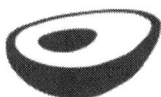

Copyright © 2016 Kasia Roberts, RN

All Rights Reserved.

Published by The Fruitful Mind

www.fruitfulbooks.com

Disclaimer

The information in this book is not to be used as medical advice. The recipes should be used in combination with guidance from your physician. Please consult your physician before beginning any diet. It is especially important for those with diabetes, and those on medications to consult with their physician before making changes to their diet.

All rights reserved. No part of this publication or the information in it may be quoted from or reproduced in any form by means such as printing, scanning, photocopying or otherwise without prior written permission of the copyright holder.

Disclaimer and Terms of Use: Effort has been made to ensure that the information in this book is accurate and complete, however, the author and the publisher do not warrant the accuracy of the information, text and graphics contained within the book due to the rapidly changing nature of science, research, known and unknown facts and internet. The Author and the publisher do not hold any responsibility for errors, omissions or contrary interpretation of the subject matter herein. This book is presented solely for motivational and informational purposes only.

Table of Contents

Introduction: Defining High Blood Pressure and How It Damages Your Body 5

The Causes of High Blood Pressure 14
    High Risk Groups 14
    Non Controllable Factors 19
    Controllable Factors 22

It Takes More than Diet - Lifestyle Modifications 24

Top 30 Superfoods 29
    1. Spinach 31
    2. Kale 33
    3. Broccoli 35
    4. Arugula 37
    5. Beets 39
    6. Garlic 41
    7. Celery 43
    8. Tomatoes 45
    9. Potatoes 47
    10. Sweet Potatoes 49
    11. Avocados 51
    12. Blueberries 53
    13. Lemons 55
    14. Kiwi Fruit 57
    15. Watermelon 59
    16. Bananas 61
    17. Pomegranate 63
    18. Beans 65
    19. Quinoa 67
    20. Flax Seed 69

21. Almonds 71
22. Pistachios 73
23. Olive Oil 75
24. Fatty Fish 77
25. Skim Milk 79
26. Low Fat Yogurt 81
27. Hibiscus 83
28. Green Tea 85
29. Coffee 87
30. Dark Chocolate 89

Heart Healthy Recipes 91
Super Green Quinoa Salad 92
Tropical Banana Salad 94
Garlic Curry Vegetables 96
Grilled Stuffed Portabella Mushrooms 98
Grilled Halibut with Watermelon Salsa 100
Chicken with Blueberry Ginger Glaze 102
Easy Bean Chili 104
Broccoli Slaw 106
Avocado Chocolate Popsicles 108
Chocolate Pomegranate Smoothie 109

Conclusion 110

Introduction: Defining High Blood Pressure and How It Damages Your Body

Elevated blood pressure is one of the largest health concerns in North America. It also happens to be one of the most widely misunderstood. Many people, even those that suffer from elevated blood pressure, fail to truly understand the causes and severity of this potentially devastating condition. To begin with, there is the misconception that only people who are overly stressed, anxious or high strung are predisposed to hypertension, or if you just lose some weight and cut out the fat and salt that hypertension will magically disappear. We can acknowledge that for some people, and I speak of a very small minority, these are the main contributing factors. For the rest of the population that suffer from high blood pressure, the cause and the control are far more complex in nature.

Considering that high blood pressure and hypertension are reaching epidemic portions in the western world, it is time to really take a good look at those factors that cause this health issue, and what ways we have the ability to control the devastating effects that high blood pressure can have on our lives. In this book, we will look at one approach for treating high blood pressure and that is through nutrition. Before we go any further, it is important to say that there isn't a single food or combination of foods in this book that will magically cure your high blood pressure. Before you even begin to look at this, you should be having conversations with your physician about the healthiest and most natural ways to treat your condition. Do not automatically shun your medications, sometimes we need them to get us started on the road to healing before we can truly begin healing ourselves.

The thirty superfoods listed in this book are here to help you control your blood pressure through diet. Each one contains nutritional components or compounds that work with your body to reduce blood pressure naturally. Whether you have suffered from high blood pressure for years, or if you are being preventative before a problem even arises, you will find sound, nutritional approaches to treating high blood pressure in the pages that follow.

To begin with, it is important that we realize that what is considered normal blood pressure, what is considered hypertension and what resides on the road between the two.

A blood pressure reading is made up of two numbers, systolic pressure, which is the "top" number, and diastolic pressure, which is the bottom number in a reading. Systolic pressure measures the amount of force in the arteries when the heart contracts, while the diastolic pressure measures the amount of force in the arteries when the heart is at rest between beats. In the past, more consideration has been given to the systolic pressure reading as an indicator or warning sign of high blood pressure, however in recent years it has been discovered that the diastolic reading can be just as important, if not more so, in recognizing and treating the potential side effects of chronic high blood pressure.

For the average person, normal blood pressure has a systolic reading of 120 mm Hg or less, and a diastolic reading of 80 mm Hg or less. Take special note of the words "or less" here. Many people go around with a typical reading of say 122/83 and think that they have low, or normal blood pressure. The truth is that while this is not severely elevated, it is above the cutoff for healthy blood pressure. It can also be an indicator that as you age, you might suffer from more severely elevated blood pressure, called hypertension, in the future. The sooner you begin acting to lower your natural blood pressure level, especially with natural remedies like the superfoods listed in this book, the sooner you begin protecting your long term health from the damaging effects of hypertension.

According to the American Heart Association, these levels are used as criteria for determining healthy, unhealthy or health crisis levels of blood pressure:

- Normal   systolic ≤ 120 mm Hg   diastolic ≤ 80 mm Hg
- Prehypertension   systolic 120-139 mm Hg   diastolic 80-89 mm Hg
- Stage 1 Hypertension   systolic 140-159 mm Hg   diastolic 90-99 mm Hg
- Stage 2 Hypertension   systolic ≥160 mm Hg   diastolic ≥100 mm Hg
- Hypertensive Crisis   systolic ≥180 mm Hg   diastolic ≥110 mm Hg

It is important to note that from minute to minute and day to day, your blood pressure reading is likely to fluctuate, especially when you factor in things such as exercise, stress and mood. However, if you are older than twenty years of age and have two to three readings where your blood pressure is in the pre hypertensive range, you should take steps to reduce it by talking to your health care provider, making healthy lifestyle modifications and introducing more of the blood pressure superfoods into your diet. If you have multiple readings in either the stage one or stage two hypertension ranges, your health care provider will likely get you started on a course of medication to help you begin to control your blood pressure. If you have a reading in the hypertensive crisis range, it is important that you seek medical attention immediately.

If you have elevated blood pressure or hypertension, you might be wondering what the health implications are. One of the most dangerous assumptions is to think that because your blood pressure isn't "that" high that you do not have to concern yourself with the effects of the additional stress on your body. When we look at blood pressure, at its most basic level, it is simply the amount of force that is being put upon your arterial walls. A certain amount of force and pressure is natural and necessary. However, when too much force, caused by even slightly elevated pressure, is applied to the arterial walls over time they begin to stretch, weaken and in some cases even become hardened. As damage occurs, the following problems can occur:

1. Vascular stretching and weakness, which can lead to the rupture of blood vessels, which can cause strokes and aneurysms.

2. Vascular scarring and plaque accumulation, which create pockets where cholesterol and blood cells can become entrapped in the veins and arteries. Once scarring and plaque buildup begin to occur, blood does not flow as freely through the veins and the heart needs to work even harder. In some cases, the scarring can be so severe, or the buildup can break away and in both cases a blockage may occur. This type of blockage leads to heart attacks.

3. Blood clots can also form in the narrowed, damaged passageways caused by high blood pressure. Just like plaque buildup, blood clots can break free and cause heart attacks and strokes.

4. Damage to your entire body, caused by lack of oxygen. Think for a moment about the important work your heart does, and how it does it. Your heart pumps freshly oxygenated blood through your body, providing every organ with the oxygen that it needs to effectively do its job.

When the passageways that your heart uses to accomplish this have been damaged by high blood pressure, your whole body suffers the consequences.

We can break this down into even simpler terms with this straightforward list of the possible health implications of untreated high blood pressure:

- Loss of eyesight
- Loss of memory
- Erectile dysfunction
- Kidney Damage
- Stroke
- Angina
- Peripheral Artery Disease
- Aortic dissection
- Atherosclerosis
- Congestive heart failure
- Coronary disease
- Heart attack
- Death

As you can see, high blood pressure is nothing to mess around with. It is a serious health condition that deserves serious consideration. You can work to take care of your body by seeing your health care provider for regular blood pressure screenings, living a life that promotes heart health, taking your medications when they are prescribed and introducing the thirty superfoods into your diet that will help naturally lower your blood pressure and possibly eliminate your need for pharmaceutical assistance in keeping your blood pressure at a healthy level.

The Causes of High Blood Pressure

The number one way of controlling high blood pressure is to find a way to prevent it from developing in the first place. However, high blood pressure and all of the contributing factors make such a simple solution difficult for most people. High blood pressure is most often not the result of a singular cause, rather a combination of factors, some inherited and some environmental, that increase your risks and determine the potential severity of your condition. We are going to break down the contributing causes of high blood pressure into three categories; high risk groups, non controllable factors, and controllable factors. Hopefully, this will help you see where you might be at a greater risk or where you can make lifestyle changes to reduce your risk.

High Risk Groups

We are not all created equal, and that is often very obvious when it comes to certain health conditions. There is a reason that most physicians are interested in your heritage and ancestral background when you see them for the first time. Factors like age, gender and ethnicity play a role in recognizing the potential development of some diseases. High blood pressure is one of those health conditions.

Women:

This one comes as a surprise to many people as it is often thought that high blood pressure is a more male centered condition. The fact is that women, especially those aged sixty or over, or after the onset of menopause, are more likely to have higher blood pressure than their same aged male counterparts. Heart disease is one of the leading causes of death in women, and it is estimated that one in three post menopausal women suffer from some form of cardiovascular disease, some of which can be attributed to high blood pressure. The hormone estrogen is thought to play a role in protecting female cardiovascular health during reproductive years and once menopause sets in, the decline in estrogen levels, combined with other factors take away that protection and leave the women more prone to developing high blood pressure and other heart related conditions.

The answer does not appear to be in estrogen supplementation after menopause, as this has not been shown to decrease the risk. Women are also at a greater risk of developing high blood pressure and potentially serious complications during pregnancy and shortly after delivery. It is extremely important to attend all of your prenatal appointments, even if you have always had completely healthy pregnancies. High blood pressure can sneak in unexpectedly. One way that women can help protect their health is by eating a diet that is low in saturated fats, high in fiber and high in superfoods.

African Americans:

African American adults have a much greater risk of developing high blood pressure than other races. In fact, it is estimated that as many as forty percent of African American adults suffer from some degree of elevated blood pressure or hypertension. There has been research in this area, but as of yet we can still only speculate at the causes of the increased risk. First of all, scientists are looking at the possibility that there is a specific gene that makes African Americans more prone to developing high blood pressure. In people with this gene, it appears that the dietary factors that can contribute to high blood pressure are amplified. For example, in most people a small amount of sodium, such as that found in a scant half teaspoon wouldn't be enough to produce immediate change in blood pressure levels.

In people identified with this gene, that same scant half teaspoon of table salt can cause a rise in blood pressure of approximately 5 mm Hg, which is quite significant. If you are African American, it is even more important that you start early and stay committed to living a lifestyle that promotes healthy blood pressure levels and make a point to stay away from foods and lifestyles that contribute to weight gain, such as high fat, high sodium foods and low levels of physical activity.

Non Controllable Factors

As frustrating as it may be, there are factors that contribute to our health that are simply beyond our control. Like many other diseases, this is also true for blood pressure levels. That are three main non controllable factors that can give you an indication of the likeliness that you will suffer from hypertension and the possible severity of your condition.

Family History:

Of the non controllable factors, your family history is possibly the most important. As was mentioned with the increased risk among African Americans, some people carry something in their genetic lineage that makes them more prone to developing high blood pressure. Take a good look at your family tree, making note of any parents, grandparents, uncles, aunts, siblings and cousins that suffer from high blood pressure. If out of a large family tree there are only a couple of people, then there is a better chance that your family history does not predispose you. However, if you notice a pattern of the disease, especially in direct lineages, then you should take extra care to live a healthy lifestyle and make regular appointments for blood pressure screenings. This is not only important for your health, but also for setting an example for the future generations. Whatever it is in your genetic makeup that predisposes you to high blood pressure can also be passed on to your children. Make an example of living a healthy lifestyle so that it becomes natural to them at a young age and not a major lifestyle shift that they need to make years down the road.

Age:

The unfortunate truth is that as we age, so does our chances for developing many health conditions, including high blood pressure. What we can do is make a point to take care of our bodies and respect them for the journey that has gotten us to this point, rather than condemn them for aging. Age can be just a number, but only if you take care of your body by living a healthy lifestyle.

Preexisting Medical Conditions:

Certain medical conditions such as heart disease and kidney disease can cause a response in the body that makes you more likely to develop high blood pressure as a secondary condition.

Controllable Factors

Here it is, the list of things you can control and use to take charge of your heart health. For a great many of us, these factors are not easy to give up or modify and can take a great commitment. However, I promise you that when you make the effort to combat high blood pressure by eliminating as many contributing factors as possible that you are working to not only extend your years, but extend the quality of each of those years. Take a hard look at this list and see where you might be able to reduce your chances of suffering the serious consequences of high blood pressure.

- Being overweight, especially with a BMI of 30 or more
- A diet that is consistently high in saturated fats and sodium
- A diet that is low in nutritional dense fruits and vegetables
- A lifestyle that lack sufficient physical exercise

- Smoking cigarettes, including inhaling secondhand smoke
- Drinking more than one to two alcoholic drinks per day
- Having uncontrollable stress

It Takes More than Diet - Lifestyle Modifications

Yes, this book is about the superfoods that you can add to your diet to prevent and treat high blood pressure, while also working to repair the damage caused by it. The hard truth is that as much as we may wish it, there is no one magic bullet for high blood pressure. There is no single pharmaceutical that can cure high blood pressure, at least not without suffering side effects and dependence upon the medication. There is no one food that can take away years of damage caused by neglect of your body and health.

Preventing and treating high blood pressure requires a multi level approach, one that you must commit to for the rest of your life. The rest of your life sounds daunting, but trust me it is worth it. Plus, for many people, once you become adjusted to the lifestyle changes, they become second nature and after a time, you simply can't imagine living your life any other way. Because of this, it seems important to make note of a few powerful lifestyle modifications that you can make, that will only amp up the healing power of the superfoods listed in this book.

• Take a look at the controllable factors in the previous chapter. How many of them are you guilty of? Giving up some of your favorite pleasures or becoming a little more active is not about punishing yourself, but rather a way to prepare yourself for a long, healthy life.

• Go to the doctor. This isn't on anyone's list of favorite things to do, but make and keep your annual appointments with your health care provider. This is vitally important for discovering and treating health related issues before they become major health obstacles.

• Find a care provider that is aligned with your beliefs. I am going to make an assumption that if you are reading this book that you are at least open to the idea that what we put into our bodies affects the output that we receive from them. You probably have an idea that as a general population, pharmaceuticals are overprescribed. There is a place for modern medicine and there is a place for the healing properties found in the natural world. Most health ailments are best treated with a combination of both. If you feel the same way, find a physician or natural health care provider that follows the same health philosophy that you do. Ask questions that are important to you and don't be afraid to walk away from a care provider that you feel uncomfortable with and who is unaligned with your beliefs.

- Get rid of stress. Ok, this is easier said than done, however, anyone can start by taking five to ten minutes a day and spending those minutes in quiet relaxing thought. At first, it may be difficult to quiet yourself and focus, it might seem like a waste of time, or your mind might be racing with thoughts of what else you should be doing. The important thing is to just start, to try and keep trying every day until you are able to spend a portion of each day devoted to quiet peacefulness. This one simple act can go a long way in reducing the effects of a stressful lifestyle on your blood pressure.

• Finally, get moving. Nothing will complement a healthy diet full of superfoods more than a consistent exercise program. You don't need to push yourself beyond your limits in order to gain the benefits of regular exercise. Just going out and moving your body is a start. Whether you can walk once around the block or run a half marathon, your fitness level isn't as important as your willingness to commit to some form of movement on a daily basis.

These lifestyle modifications, combined with a diet full of the superfoods listed in the next chapter are major steps to living a life free of high blood pressure and a life that is not dependent upon a cabinet full of pharmaceuticals. The power to heal, even with the help of a physician, is within yourself.

TOP 30
SUPERFOODS

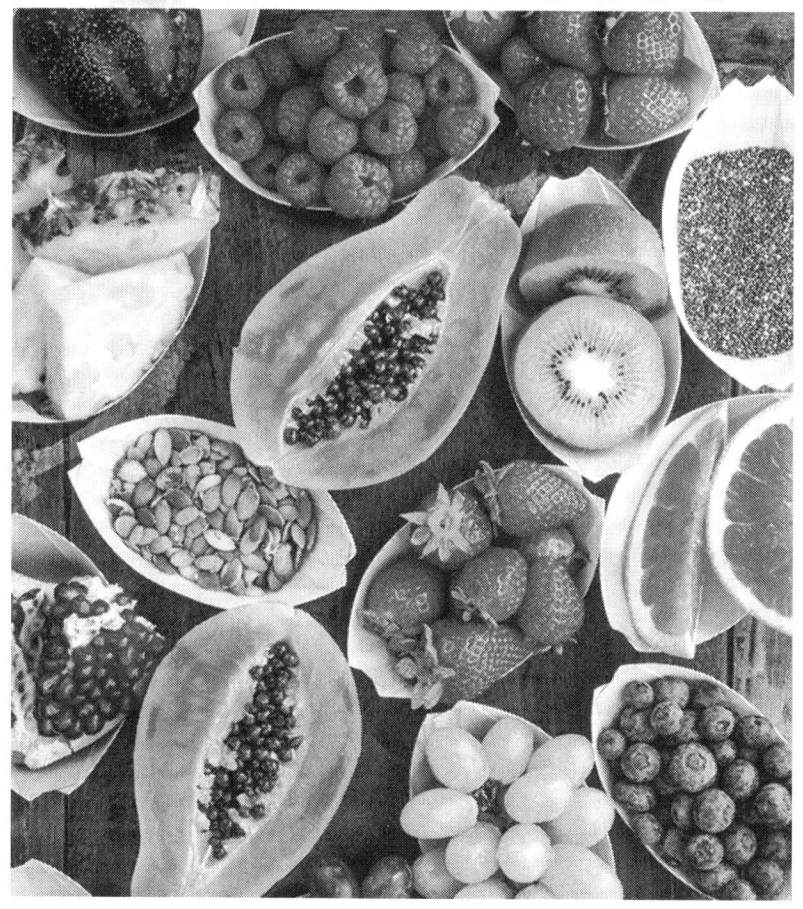

1.Spinach

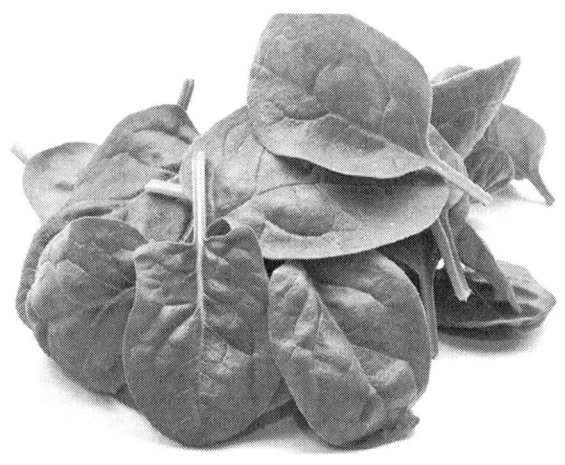

Vegetables that are rich in nitrates, such as spinach, have a powerful effect on lowering blood pressure. A recent study published in the New England Journal of Medicine noted that nitrate supplementation was effective at lowering diastolic levels in the participants. You do not need supplementation though to receive these benefits. Just add crisp, nutrient dense spinach to your diet and to achieve the same results. Spinach is low in calories, versatile and contains balanced portions of anti oxidants and protein, which all work together to boost your body's ability to lower and maintain a healthy blood pressure.

Getting it in your diet: Spinach is easy to add into your daily diet. It can be added to sandwiches; sautéed vegetables, as a topping for potatoes, a hearty salad base, and if you are in any way offended by the taste, simply add it to a smoothie with sweet fruits to balance the flavor.

2. Kale

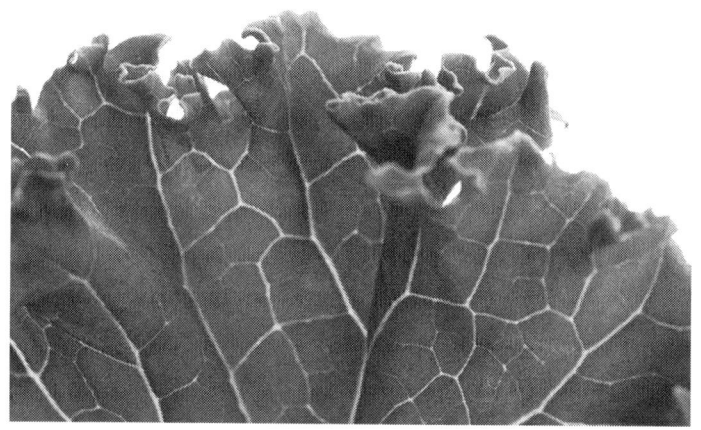

Like the above mentioned spinach, kale is extremely high in nutritional content, bite after delicious bite. Kale has the additional benefit of a more diverse and unique nutritional profile that includes ample amounts of magnesium along with other nutrients and antioxidants. Magnesium works with potassium to boost its blood pressure lowering effects. Given the fact that the average western diet is deficient in potassium, the extra magnesium in kale goes a long way in protecting the health of those who eat it. Kale is also a good source for vitamin C, making it a true superfood.

Getting it in your diet: If you are not familiar with it, kale can be a little intimidating at first. After all, isn't it supposed to be a garnish? Sure, a truly edible and delicious garnish! Depending upon your preferences, kale can be served raw or cooked. Many people like to drizzle kale with a little olive oil and bake it in the oven to create kale chips. It can also be chopped up and added to dips, soups, salads and smoothies for a quick boost of nutrition.

3. Broccoli

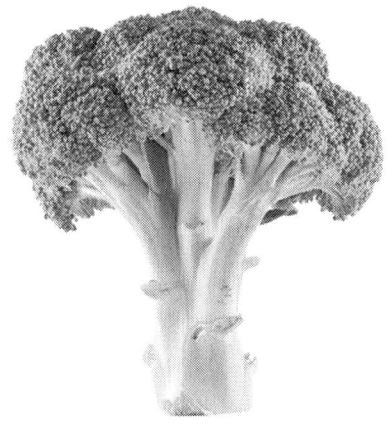

As a child, you may have constantly been reminded to eat your broccoli. What you probably didn't know at the time was that you were also protecting your long term health by eating the "little trees". Broccoli, and other cruciferous vegetables contain a compound that produces a metabolite by the name of sulforaphane, that has been shown to reduce blood pressure in studies. Broccoli is also a rich source of potassium, magnesium and calcium; a power trio for lowering blood pressure. It doesn't matter if you eat it cooked or raw, this versatile vegetable will improve your health while improving the quality of your meal.

Getting it in your diet: Broccoli is the perfect vegetable snack, holding up well on its own or a light, healthy dip. It is also perfect when steamed to tender perfection or added into just about any dish you can imagine. Try adding a handful, or more, of broccoli into your next soup, casserole or topping for a potato.

4. Arugula

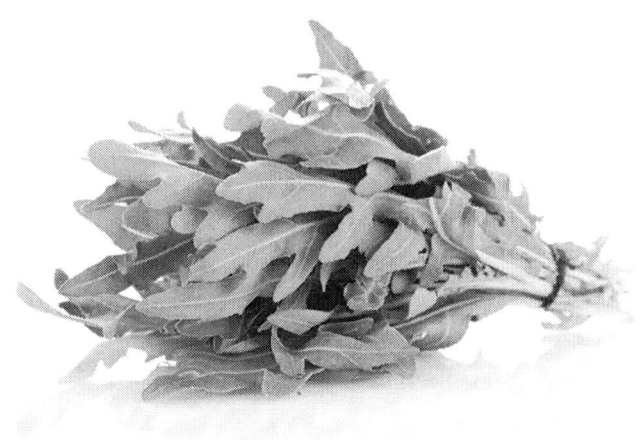

Arugula has gained popularity in recent years, and who can blame the culinary world for promoting this superfood? It is snappy and peppery, adding just the right texture and flavor to salads and sandwiches. With roots in the cruciferous family, it shares the intense nutritional composition, including the metabolite sulforaphane. In addition, arugula is also rich in vitamins A, C, K, B6 and magnesium, potassium and calcium. It helps to lower blood pressure and improve overall vascular function in the body.

Getting it in your diet: Arugula, once a little more obscure, is not readily available in most amply stocked produce sections. The best way to add arugula into your diet is through adding it to your salads for unsurpassed flavor. It also makes a nice additive as a green for sandwiches and even a lighter, healthier pizza.

5. Beets

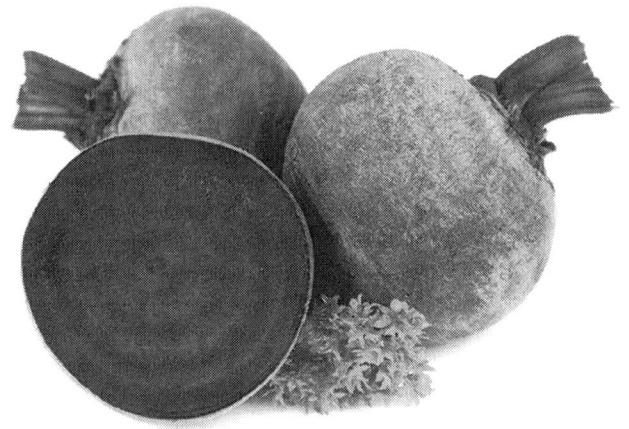

Like spinach, beets are also good sources of nitrates. You might be thinking to yourself that your doctor, or the media, has advised you to avoid nitrate rich foods, like hot dogs, lunch meat and bacon, but no one has mentioned beets. This is because there is more than one type of nitrate complex and the ones you have been told to avoid are no comparison to the healthy nitrate complex found in beets. The nitrates in beets can be converted into nitric oxide, a compound that can actually reduce blood pressure in just a matter of hours by widening the blood vessels and thus improving blood flow. The benefits of beets can be obtained through consuming the root or drinking beet juice.

Getting it in your diet: Try adding some beet juice to your next smoothie or soup. When roasted with a little olive oil, beet roots make a nice, mildly sweet addition to almost any meal, including salads and stews.

6. Garlic

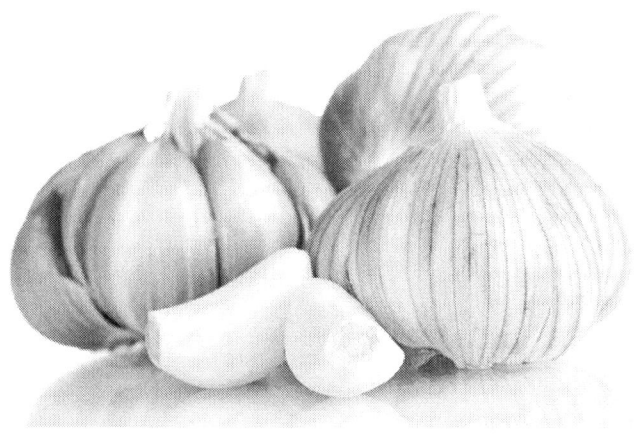

Do you like your food with lots of flavor? If so, then garlic is the perfect superfood for you. Throughout the world, cultures use garlic to enhance their traditional dishes. Today, we have such a love affair with garlic, that you can find recipes such as Forty Clove Chicken, or Extreme Garlic Sauce that not only highlight the flavor of garlic, but make it the center of the dish. Garlic has an effect that goes beyond what it does for your taste buds, and your breath. Garlic has been shown to significantly reduce blood pressure levels when consumed regularly over time. The active, blood pressuring reducing compound in garlic is a sulphur called allicin. When the garlic is crushed, this compound is released and works wonders. Just one to two cloves of garlic a day can be as effective in lowering blood pressure as some medications over time.

Getting it in your diet: How do you get garlic into your diet? Add it to everything! Try it raw, in small amounts, sautéed or if the sharpness puts you off, try it roasted to bring out the slightly sweet and nutty undertones.

7. Celery

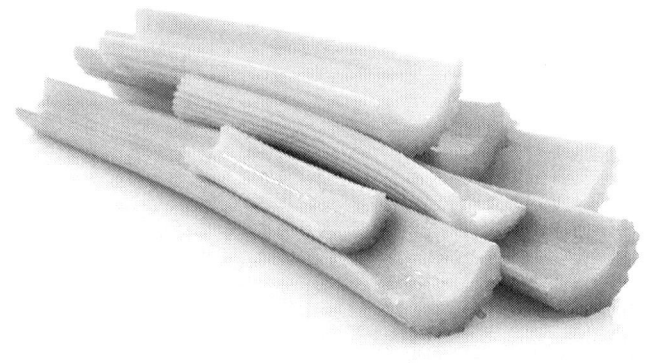

Some superfoods are the stars of the show, while others are the stagehands, behind the scenes working unnoticed. Celery is like a stagehand of the superfoods. Celery on its own, celery contains phthalides which relax the arterial walls and help promote healthy circulation. However, most people might find it difficult to consume enough celery, approximately three to four stalks, daily to reap the most benefits. If you love celery, then crunch away. However, if that amount makes you apprehensive, think of all of the ways that you can add celery into your diet to help boost the blood pressure lowering potential of other super foods while providing you with a well balanced nutritional profile with its high fiber, magnesium and potassium content.

Getting it in your diet: Enjoy it raw as a snack with walnuts or in a salad. Or, you can sauté it and add it to any dish, including a blood pressure friendly stir fry.

8. Tomatoes

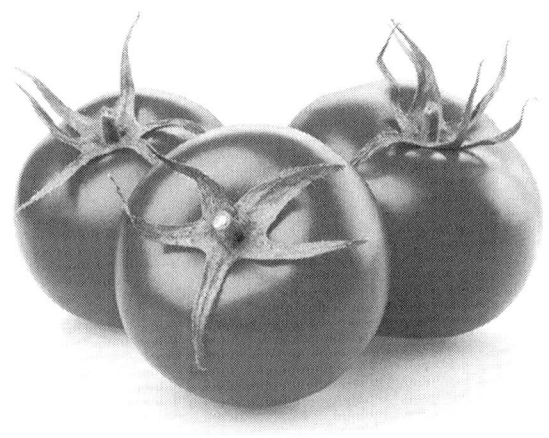

If you are looking for a food that will help lower your blood pressure, that you probably already have in your diet, the answer is the tomato. We consume tomatoes in so many ways, like pasta sauce, pizza sauce, tomato paste based sauces, ketchup, and straight from the garden. Tomatoes are good sources of lycopene, which has been shown to be as effective at reducing high blood pressure as some low dose medications. Just twenty-five milligrams of lycopene is enough to produce an effect. How much juicy tomato goodness is that? Chances are you already consume it on some days. Just one half cup of tomato juice or sauce has close to the recommended amount. Switch out your morning beverage for a glass of tomato juice and you have just started your day in the best way possible.

Getting it in your diet: You can eat tomatoes raw, in juices or cooked. However, keep in mind that many premade tomato sauces are also high in sodium and/or sugar, which are two substances that can be counterproductive to your blood pressure lowering efforts. Read labels, or better yet, make a simple sauce or tomato juice from scratch in your own kitchen.

9. Potatoes

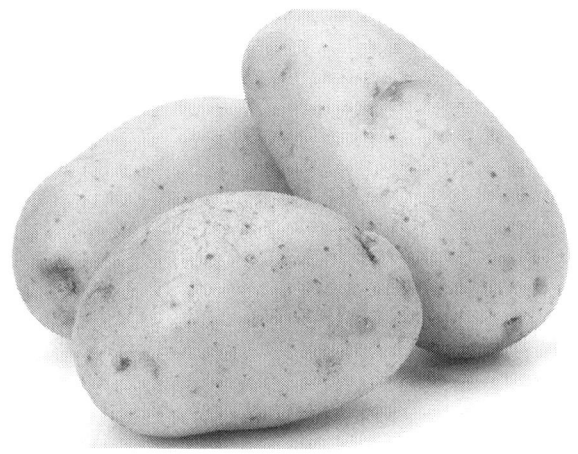

Here we are talking about the plain, old fashioned white potato. You might have heard that there really isn't any nutritional benefit to potatoes, and that the starchy carbohydrates add a negative health effect that outweighs any good. The truth is that for heart and blood pressure health, nothing could be further from the truth. Potassium is key for proper health. When your body is depleted of potassium, you automatically retain extra sodium. What does excess sodium equate to? You got it, high blood pressure. By keeping potassium in the body at higher levels, you will naturally eliminate the excess sodium in your body. This means that high potassium foods, such as the potato, are important for your blood pressure lowering diet.

Getting it in your diet: Keep away from the fry oils and you will be fine. Try a potato, baked, steamed or even mashed as long as you go easy on the butter, or skip it altogether. There are lots of healthy ways to top a baked potato, many of them are included in this list!

10. Sweet Potatoes

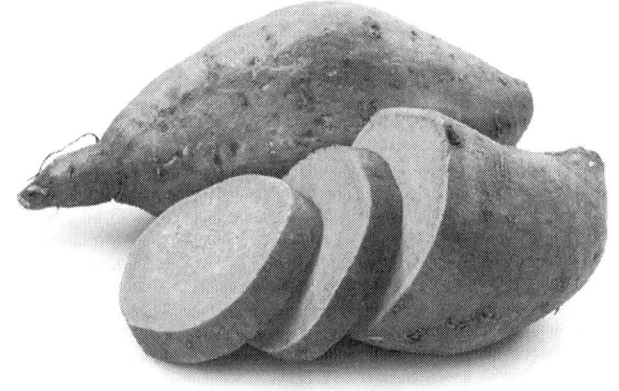

While the standard potato is great for lowering blood pressure, the sweet potato is even better. This is because sweet potatoes are nutritionally dense and pack a powerful potassium punch. In addition to this, sweet potatoes have a flavor that is naturally richer, and they are very filling, making them highly satisfying, even to the point that they can stand alone as the star of a meal.

Getting it in your diet: Bake them, mash them, roast them, dare I say even fry them in a heart healthy oil. Season them with savory herbs and spices or spice them up with just a bit of maple or brown sugar. Sweet potatoes can be topped and served as a main course, or served as a side dish.

11. Avocados

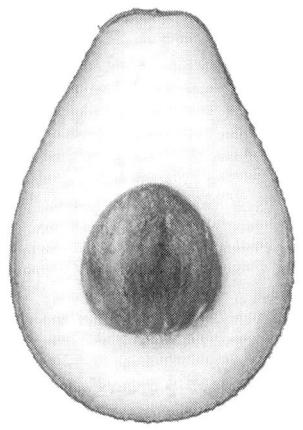

Chances are pretty good that you have heard of all of the heart healthy benefits that are packed into just avocado. In fact, many people, including those on low carbohydrate diets and those who suffer from inflammatory health conditions, consider the mighty avocado to be one of their primary daily foods. Avocados contain heart healthy oil and a perfect portion of fat and protein. However, they are also rich in potassium and in combination with their healthy fat content, this makes them the perfect food lowering blood pressure.

Getting it in your diet: The most famous way of eating avocado is probably guacamole, which you can dress up in just about any style you desire. However, avocado is delicious in its simplicity when sliced and added to salads and sandwiches. You can also try an avocado stuffed with tuna salad or egg for a high protein, blood pressure lowering snack or light lunch.

12. Blueberries

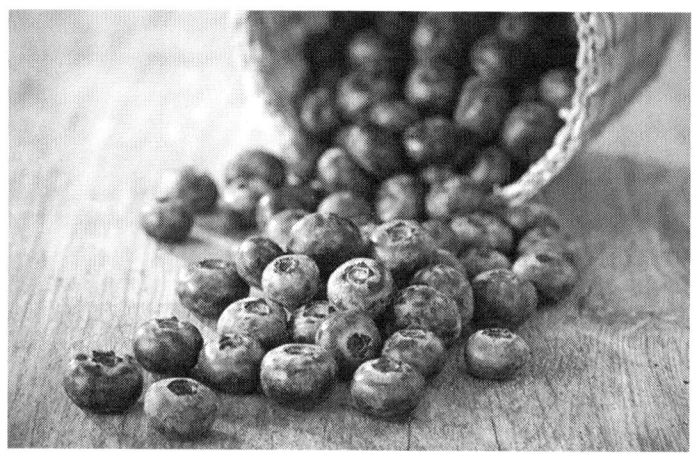

What if instead of popping a pill in your mouth, you could pop in sweet, juicy blueberries to help reduce your blood pressure? While completely replacing your blood medication with blueberries is not advisable, increasing your intake of the little purplish gems could help prevent blood pressure levels from elevating in the first place and reduce the risk of severe hypertension. Blueberries contain flavonoids, which produce nitric oxide, that magical blood vessel softening compound. The relaxation of the walls of the blood vessels reduces the stress placed upon them, and thus reduces blood pressure and the possibility that elevated blood pressure might be a future health issue for you. It turns out this is especially true for post menopausal women who were the subject of a recent study. The women in the study, with an average age of fifty-five years, showed a reduction in blood pressure levels after just eight weeks of daily blueberry consumption.

Getting it in your diet: Fresh is best, especially when tossed onto salads and into smoothies. However, this little berry only burst more with flavor when cooked and can be the center of unexpectedly savory sauces.

13. Lemons

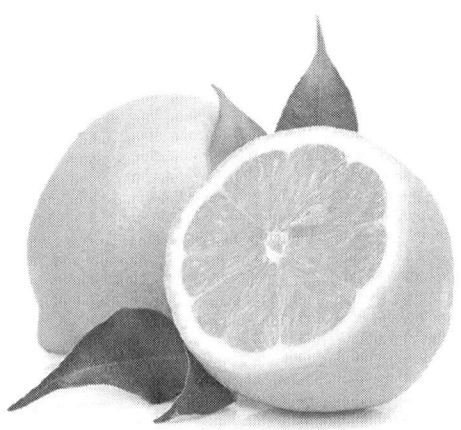

This pleasant citrus is high in vitamin C and helps to reduce the effects of free radicals in the body. This can include negative effects to your cardiovascular health, including hypertension. Lemons help to make the arterial walls become softer, less rigid and reduce the stress placed upon them by a chronic hypertensive state.

Getting it in your diet: Just give it a squeeze. Keep fresh lemons cut up and ready to squeeze into your favorite drinks, or over seafood, chicken, desserts and salads. For an especially soothing remedy, try a little lemon in a nice warm cup of water or your favorite tea.

14. Kiwi Fruit

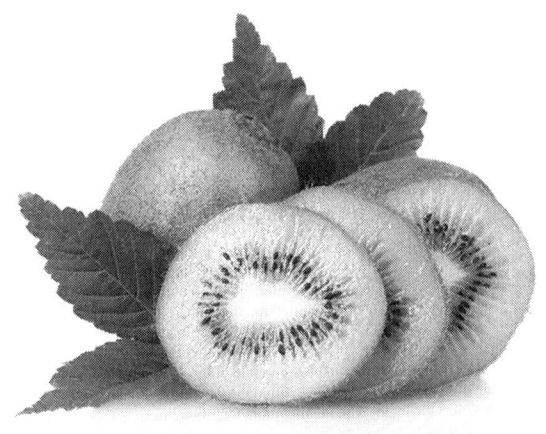

Another surprising addition to the anti hypertension remedy list. Kiwis surprise the palate by being both slightly tart and sweet at the same time, and when at their peak of sweet juiciness, they simply can't be beat. Add to this that kiwis are rich in the antioxidant, lutien, and you not only have a perfect snack, but also the perfect remedy for lowering blood pressure. Studies show that in a group of people aged over fifty, adding kiwi to the diet daily had played a role in the overall reduction of blood pressure levels.

Getting it in your diet: If you aren't familiar with kiwi, now is the time to get acquainted. Once you strip the fruit of its furry brown skin, you will reveal a green, juicy nugget of sweetness. Peel it and slice it to serve with yogurt for a sweet treat. It can also be added to smoothies, salads and cottage cheese for a quick snack.

15. Watermelon

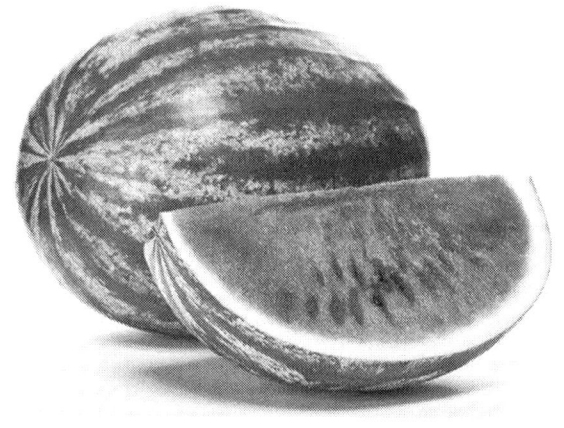

If you have thought of watermelon as only an occasional summer treat, it is time to rethink your image and consider adding it to your grocery list year round. For starters, watermelon is hydrating and keeping your body properly hydrated is one of the most important things you can do to promote overall good health. Secondly, watermelon contains a compound called citrulline, which leads to the production of nitric acid. At this point, the story of nitric acid might be familiar to you. Nitric acid helps to soften the arterial walls, widen them and reduce the stress that is placed upon them. This all adds up to one thing: lower blood pressure.

Getting it in your diet: Begin by slicing open a watermelon any time of year. Secondly, try a new approach to the old favorite by serving it grilled with fresh mint, or as an addition to a nice cold glass of water or homemade lemonade.

16. Bananas

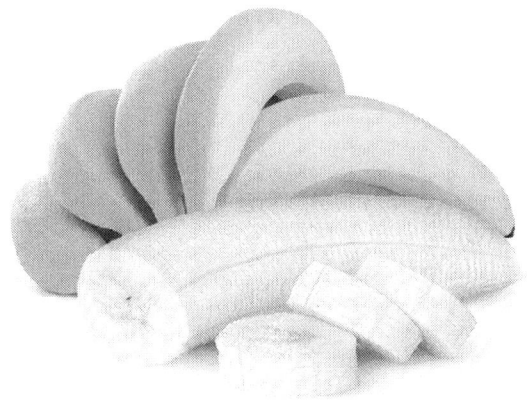

The banana is possibly one of the most common, familiar and comfortable food on this list. It is one that is given to babies as one of their very first foods, and it is one that is enjoyed throughout a lifetime either fresh or as an addition to meals and desserts. Bananas rank among the blood pressure super foods because they are incredibly rich in potassium, a mineral that helps the body balance the effects of sodium in the body and naturally regulates blood pressure. Eating one to two bananas a day is enough to supply your body with enough potassium to help reduce blood pressure in as little as eight weeks.

Getting it in your diet: You can find bananas at most any grocery store, farmers market or even gas stations and convenience stores. They are one of the most beloved fruits. Most of the time, the best way to enjoy a banana is probably straight from the skin, but you can also add them to baked goods and smoothies for incredible flavor and texture.

17. Pomegranate

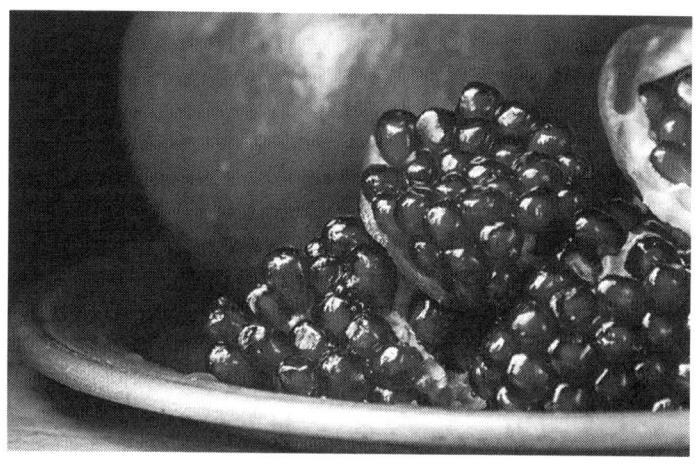

The pomegranate is a mysterious and attractive fruit. You cut it open and these sweet and tart little gleaming gems just pour forth. Making headlines in recent years, the pomegranate has become known as a healthy powerhouse. The pomegranate is a natural ACE inhibitor, which is the exact type of medication that many people with hypertension are already taking. The natural compounds in the pomegranate protect cardiovascular health, and are anti-inflammatory in nature. Pomegranates are not only a superfood for your blood pressure, but for promoting good health all around.

Getting it in your diet: The best way to consume pomegranate while gaining the most benefit is through the sweet and tart juice. Typically, when you talk about drinking any fruit juice for health benefits, you need to consume a large amount to produce any results. With pomegranate juice, just a couple of ounces a day for eight weeks is enough to show improvement in the condition of hypertension.

18. Beans

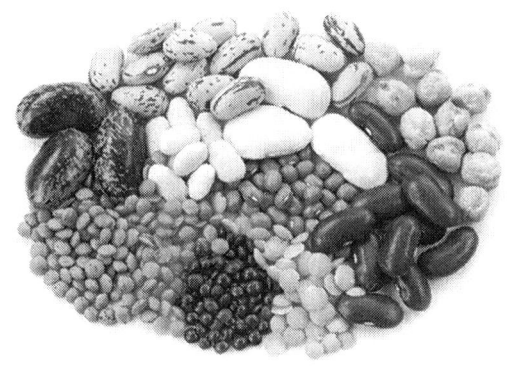

A variety of beans such as pinto, kidney, white, lima and navy beans are great for heart health. To begin with, beans contain fiber which is important for both the digestive and cardiovascular systems. In addition to this, beans are rich in potassium which is an absolute must in supporting healthy blood pressure levels.

Getting it in your diet: You can feature them as the star of the show, or add them to just about any dish you can imagine. The wide variety of beans and the different ways you can prepare them and the range of flavors that you can pair them with mean that you can eat beans several times a week and never have to worry about boredom.

19. Quinoa

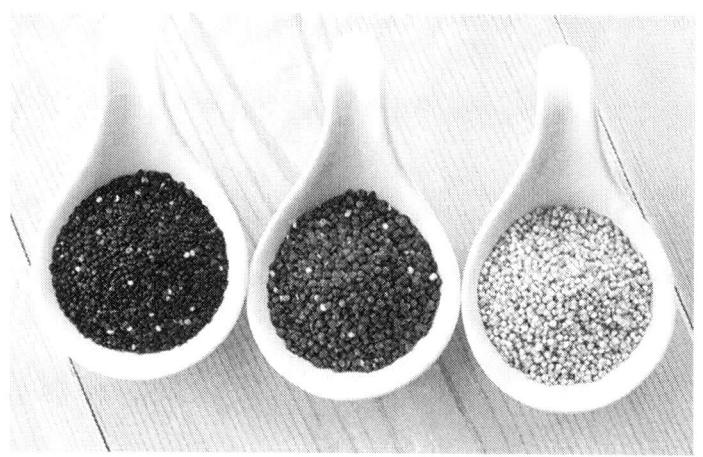

If you have ever heard the terms "super grain" or the "mother of all grains", chances are it was in reference to quinoa. Considered one of the worlds healthiest foods, quinoa has twice as much fiber and potassium as other grains and it is also rich in magnesium. This combination makes it an absolute must to add to your superfood pantry to fight hypertension.

Getting it in your diet: Quinoa can be prepared in either sweet or savory recipes, meaning you can enjoy it for breakfast, lunch, dinner or even dessert. Keep cooked quinoa on hand to add to your favorite salad, soup or hot morning breakfast.

20. Flax Seed

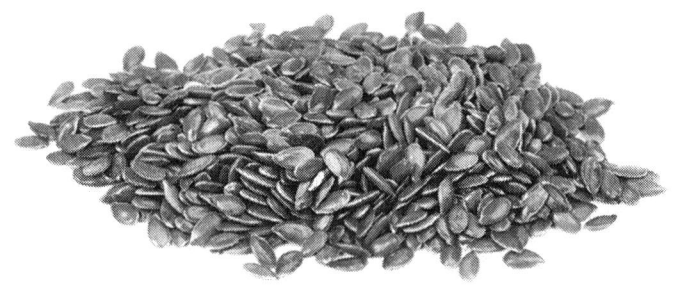

Flax seed is such a powerful antihypertensive that the American Heart Association even promotes it in addition to a heart healthy, blood pressure lowering diet. Flax seed is high in fiber and rich in Omega 3 fatty acids, which are the good fats that promote healing and protection of cardiovascular health. A study showed that after a period of six months, people who had added flax seed to their diet showed marked improvements in lowering their blood pressure over their counterparts in the study who did not add flax seed to their diets.

Getting it in your diet: The best way to get more flax seed into your diet is to sprinkle it on almost anything. It can be added to smoothies, breakfast cereal, yogurt, salads and added to baked goods for extra crunch and nutritional value.

21. Almonds

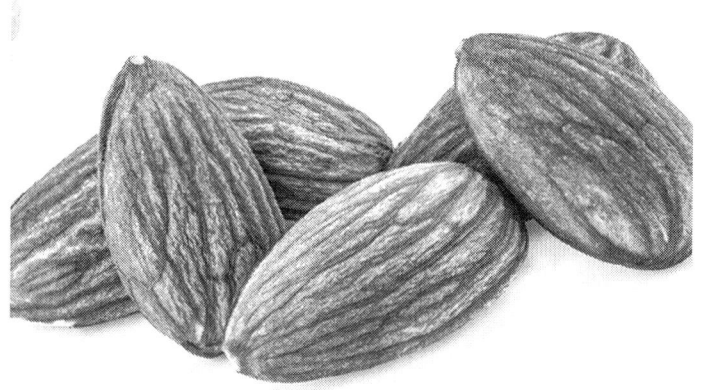

If you are looking for a heart healthy snack, you need look no further than the mighty almond. While small in size, the almond packs a big punch when it comes to flavor, texture, versatility and nutrition. About two ounces of almonds, provides ten percent of the daily recommended amount of potassium, which is vital for blood pressure regulation.

Getting it in your diet: An ounce of almonds is considered a snack portion, however if you reach for prepackaged snack size almonds, chances are you will get at least two ounces, rather than one. While a little higher in calories than some snacks, the nutritional benefit can easily outweigh the extra calories, just make sure that you get the unsalted variety. Almonds can also be added to cereal, yogurt, ground as a flour and even used as a coating when baking foods.

22. Pistachios

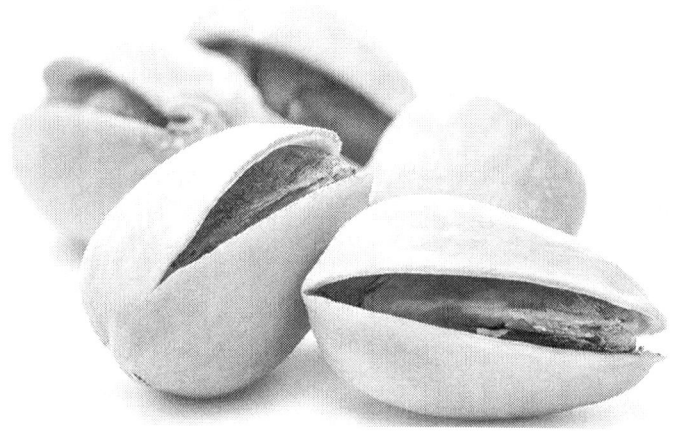

You may have heard about the powerful heart healthy effects of walnuts and almonds, which are listed above as one of our heart healthy superfoods. However, did you know that there is another nut, that potentially is even more powerful at combating high blood pressure and high cholesterol than either the almond or the walnut? This super nut is the pistachio. According to a review that was presented in the American Journal of Clinical Nutrition, pistachios, with high amounts of phytosterols and monounsaturated fatty acids prove to be effective at reducing blood pressure levels in, especially in people with type II diabetes.

Getting it in your diet: Add a handful of pistachios to your salad, cereal or snack bag. Their unique flavor and addictive crunch make them an enjoyable addition to even meat or seafood dishes.

23. Olive Oil

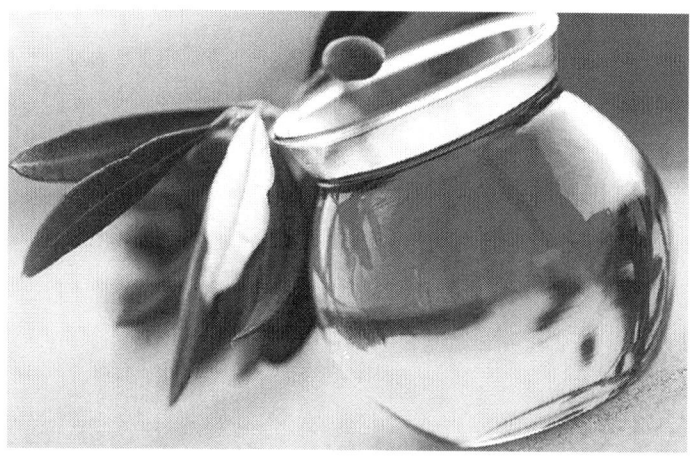

There is a general mindset that fat is bad. The truth is that sometimes, fat is very good especially when it is coming from a source such as olive oil. Olive oil is rich in polyphenols, which protect LDL cholesterol from free radicals and oxidation. By preventing the oxidation of LDL cholesterol, olive oil prevents the hardening of the arterial walls, making it so that the blood can flow through freely without excess resistance. Over the course of one study, patients who replaced other fats in their diet with olive oil were able to reduce the need for blood pressure medication by approximately half. Those are some pretty powerful statistics, especially considering how available olive oil is and how easily it can be incorporated into the average diet.

Getting it in your diet: First of all, make sure that you are getting one hundred percent pure olive oil. Many companies dilute their olive oil and sell it as a blend. You will get the most benefit from olive oil when you avoid the blends and go for the pure oil. Depending on what you plan to use it for, there are several options available. The more purely you intend to use it, as a dressing for example, the more you should favor extra virgin varieties because their flavor will be better suited for that use.

24. Fatty Fish

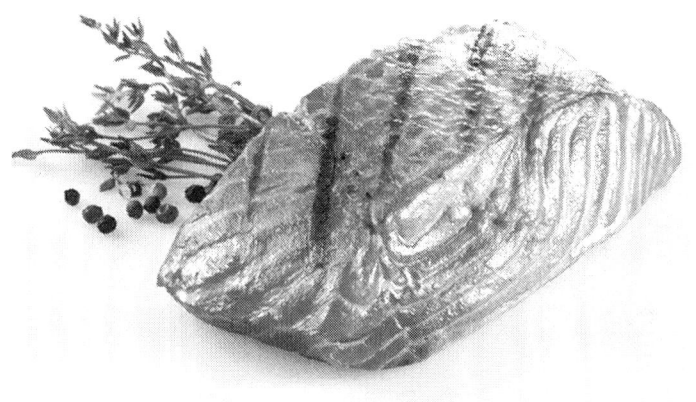

The omega 3 fatty acids found in fatty fish, such as salmon, mackerel and sardines, are excellent for promoting overall cardiovascular health, including keeping your blood pressure in check. Throughout this list of superfoods, you find a lot foods that can be snacks or subtle additions to your diet. Only a few of the superfoods are ones that can make up the filling, protein rich main part of the meal. Fatty fish is an exceptional star in this list of superfoods. The American Heart Association recommends eating fatty fish two times per week, unless you have a medical condition that limits the amount of fatty fish that you should consume.

Getting it in your diet: Grill it, steam it, bake it and enjoy it an almost unlimited variety of ways. Cook it with olive oil and top it with lemon juice and an almond or pistachio crust for an even more powerful superfood.

25. Skim Milk

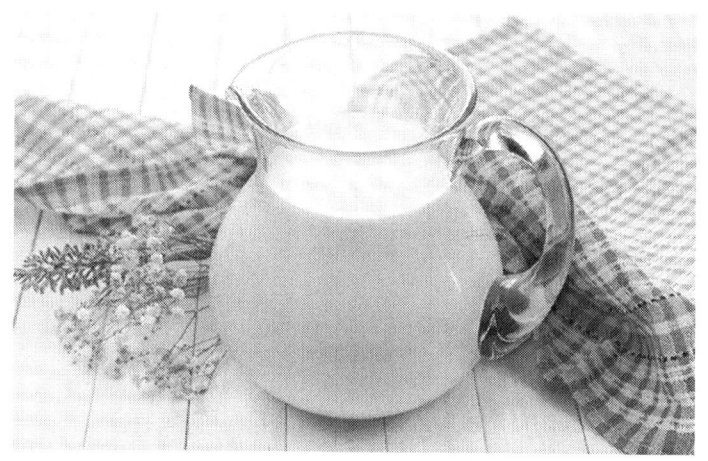

A glass of day keeps the blood pressure medication away, or at least helps your medication out. Just one glass of skim milk has enough calcium, magnesium and potassium to provide you with enough heart healthy benefits to help you control and manage your hypertension. Studies show that people who drink one glass of milk a day have a lesser incidence of hypertension years into the future, and over a period of time, drinking skim milk daily can reduce the dependence on blood pressure lowering medications.

Getting it in your diet: Even if you don't really care for the taste of milk, it is easy to add eight ounces a day into your diet through smoothies or by adding a healthy drink powder into it and making a heart healthy milk shake.

26. Low Fat Yogurt

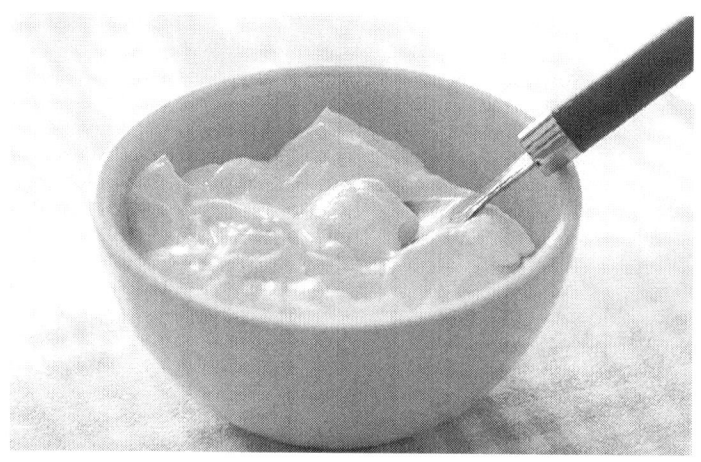

For many of the same reasons that skim milk is a superfood, high calcium, magnesium and potassium levels, yogurt also ranks among the thirty best foods for controlling blood pressure, especially in women. A study showed that women, who consumed at least five servings of low fat yogurt per week, demonstrated a twenty percent reduction in the risk of hypertension. It is very possible that this effect does not pertain strictly to women, it is just that women are more likely to consume more low fat yogurt than the typical man during the week. So, male or female it doesn't matter, eat up!

Getting it in your diet: Cool and creamy, low fat yogurt is perfect for breakfast, snack or dessert. Instead of buying sweetened and flavored varieties which can be high in sugar, try opting for plain low fat yogurt and flavor it yourself with fresh fruits, nuts, honey and grains.

27. Hibiscus

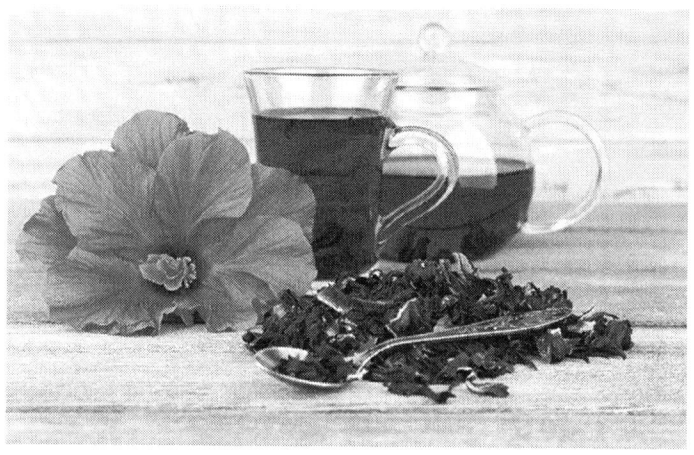

Hibiscus is a beautiful flower that is native to warm and subtropical areas. Aside from its aesthetic contribution, the dried hibiscus flower makes a mild floral tea that is favored all over the world. What some of the world already knows is that hibiscus tea isn't just for enjoyment; in some countries it is used as a medicinal remedy for blood pressure and research shows that two weeks of drinking hibiscus tea can be just as effective at lowering blood pressure as some commonly prescribed medications. They key to using hibiscus to lower your blood pressure is to be consistent. The results last only as long as you keep up your daily tea routine.

Getting it in your diet: Make a ritual out of it. Choose a time of day to sit quietly and enjoy a cup a hibiscus tea, either hot or cold.

28. Green Tea

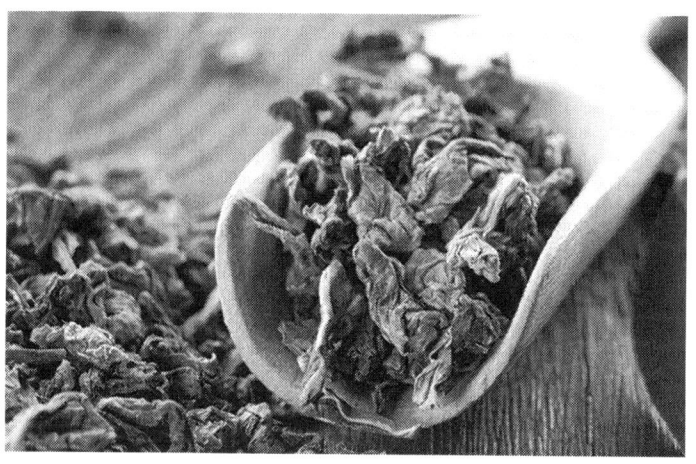

Green tea contains polyphenols, one of the most powerful of which is a catechin by the name of epigallocatechin-3-gallate. This catechin makes green tea a super antioxidant and super anti-inflammatory, two properties which serve well to support healthy blood pressure levels. Several studies have shown that just twelve weeks of daily green tea consumption showed improvements in the both systolic and diastolic blood pressure levels in people with hypertension.

Getting it in your diet: You can brew green tea and drink it hot or cold, however it can also be infused into a number of dishes including soups and desserts to add a mild and slightly grassy flavor component.

29. Coffee

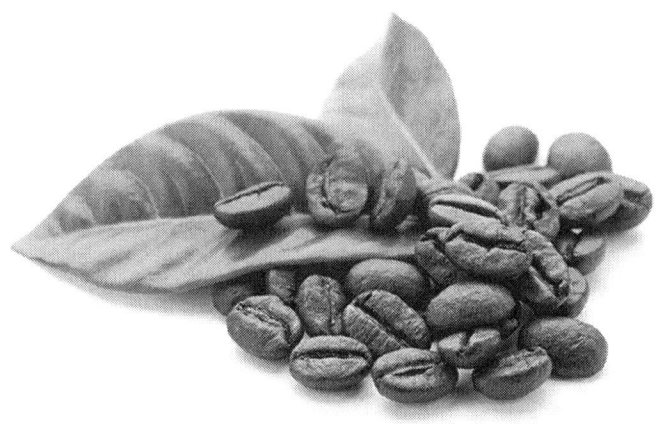

You might be surprised to find this one on this list since caffeinated beverages are known for their blood pressure raising properties. The thing is that coffee, like certain teas, contains flavonoids which actually help to relax arterial walls and promote easier blood flow. The key to coffee being a superfood for lowering blood pressure all resides in the word moderation. One cup of caffeinated coffee per day is enough to gain the heart health benefits without the caffeine content making your blood pressure worse.

Getting it in your diet: One cup a day, hot or cold, black or with skim milk is the perfect way to gain the heart healthy benefits of coffee. You can also use coffee in baking and it is a surprisingly perfect addition to a spicy chili or rich roast.

30. Dark Chocolate

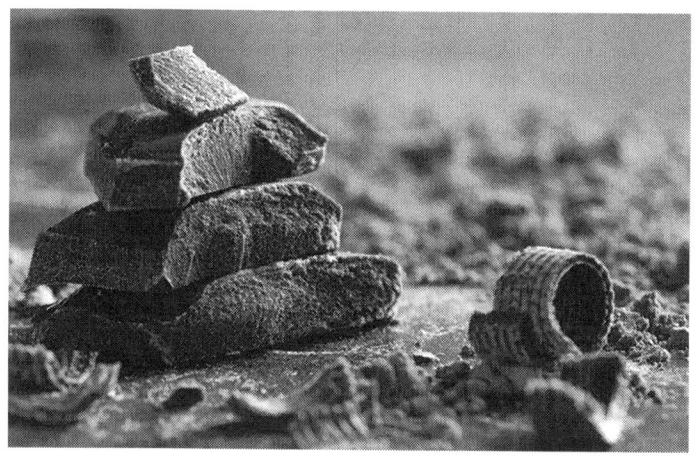

We have saved the most decadent superfood for last. Chocolate lovers celebrate that rich, indulgent dark chocolate is good for your health. In a study of over one thousand participants that ate an ounce of dark chocolate per day, all of them showed a lowering of blood pressure levels. This result was even more noticeable in those participants that actually suffered from hypertension. The key here is that it must be dark chocolate, at least sixty to seventy percent cocoa to really get the benefits. So, skip the average candy bar and stroll over to the grown up candy section where you will find luscious dark chocolate just waiting to be part of your heart healthy diet.

Getting it in your diet: A one ounce square a day is the perfect amount. You can eat it plain or add it to a few other blood pressure lowering foods, for example a selection of blueberries, pomegranate, pistachio and dark chocolate, a perfect compliment.

Heart Healthy Recipes

Now you have this list of thirty superfoods for high blood pressure, but aren't quite sure how to begin incorporating them into your diet. Here we provide you with ten recipes to get you started. These recipes will not only make a difference in how energetic and vibrant you feel, but also help you see how easy it is to eat these superfoods in creative and tasty ways.

Super Green Quinoa Salad

Ingredients:

4 cups fresh spinach, torn

1 cup kale, torn

1 cup arugula, torn

1 cup quinoa, cooked

½ cup pomegranate seeds

½ cup pistachios, chopped

¼ cup olive oil

2 tablespoons fresh lemon juice

1 tablespoon Dijon mustard

1 tablespoon fresh thyme

1 teaspoon coarse ground black pepper

Directions:

In a bowl, combine the spinach, kale, arugula and quinoa. Toss to mix.

In a separate bowl combine the olive oil, lemon juice, Dijon mustard, thyme and black pepper. Whisk together until well blended.

Drizzle the dressing over the greens and toss to coat.

Sprinkle in the pomegranate seeds and pistachios right before serving and toss gently to mix.

Tropical Banana Salad

Ingredients:

4 cups fresh spinach leaves

2 cups bananas, chopped in large pieces

2 cups kiwi, diced

1 tablespoon jalapeno pepper, diced

½ cup cucumber, peeled and diced

½ cup red bell pepper, diced

2 tablespoons olive oil

1 tablespoon champagne vinegar

2 tablespoons lime juice

1 teaspoon lime zest

1 teaspoon local honey

2 cloves garlic, crushed and minced

Directions:

In a bowl combine the olive oil, champagne vinegar, lime juice, lime zest, honey and garlic. Whisk together until well blended.

In another bowl combine the banana, kiwi, cucumber, and red bell pepper. Toss gently to mix.

Place the spinach onto serving plates and top with a scoop of the banana mixture.

Drizzle the dressing over the banana mixture and spinach before serving. Serve with extra dressing on the side, if desired.

Garlic Curry Vegetables

Ingredients:

2 tablespoons olive oil

2 cups sweet potatoes, cut into small cubes

4 cloves garlic, crushed and minced

½ cup onion, diced

1 cup chickpeas, cooked or canned and drained

2 cups broccoli florets

1 cup low sodium chicken or vegetable stock

2 cups low fat coconut milk

1 tablespoon red curry paste

1 teaspoon lime zest

4 cups fresh spinach, torn

1 teaspoon fresh ground black pepper

2 cups quinoa, cooked

1 tablespoon fresh lemongrass, chopped

Directions:

Heat the olive oil in a large, deep skillet over medium heat. Add the sweet potatoes and sauté for 4-5 minutes.

Add the garlic and onions and cook, stirring frequently for an additional 3-4 minutes.

Add the chickpeas, broccoli and chicken or vegetable stock. Cook, stirring frequently for 3-5 minutes.

Combine the coconut milk, red curry paste and lime zest. Pour the mixture into the skillet and bring to a low boil. Reduce the heat, cover and let simmer for 5-7 minutes.

Add the spinach and let cook just until wilted.

Season with black pepper as desired and serve with cooked quinoa, garnished with fresh lemongrass.

Grilled Stuffed Portabella Mushrooms

Ingredients:

4 large portabella mushroom caps

2 tablespoons olive oil

1 cup tomatoes, diced

1 cup green bell pepper, diced

2 cloves garlic, crushed and minced

1 tablespoon lemon juice

½ cup unsalted walnuts, chopped

¼ cup fresh basil, chopped

2 cups quinoa, cooked

¼ cup fresh grated parmesan cheese

Directions:

Preheat an indoor or outdoor grill over medium heat.

Brush the mushroom caps with one tablespoon of the olive oil. Place the caps on the grill, gill side down and grill for 2-3 minutes before turning over and grilling an additional 2-3 minutes. Remove and set aside.

Add the remaining oil to a skillet over medium heat.

Add the tomatoes, bell pepper, garlic and lemon juice to the skillet and sauté for 3-5 minutes, or until the peppers are crisp tender. Remove the contents from the skillet and transfer to a bowl.

To the vegetables add in the walnuts, basil and quinoa. Toss to mix.

Add equal amounts of the mixture into the center of the mushroom caps and top with fresh grated parmesan cheese.

Place the caps back on the grill and cook until warmed through with the cheese slightly melted on top.

Grilled Halibut with Watermelon Salsa

Ingredients:

1 lb. halibut fillets

1 teaspoon black pepper

½ teaspoon chili powder

1 tablespoon olive oil

1 cup watermelon, diced

½ cup fresh pineapple, diced

½ cup red onion, diced

1 tablespoon jalapeno pepper

¼ cup fresh cilantro

Directions:

In a bowl combine the watermelon, pineapple, onion, jalapeno pepper and cilantro.

Cover and place in the refrigerator for at least 30 minutes.

Season the halibut with black pepper and chili powder.

Add the olive oil to a skillet over medium heat.

Place the fish in the skillet and cook 5-7 minutes per side, or until cooked through.

Remove from the skillet and top with the chilled watermelon salsa.

Chicken with Blueberry Ginger Glaze

Ingredients:

1 lb. boneless, skinless chicken breast

1 tablespoon olive oil

½ teaspoon onion powder

½ teaspoon black pepper

1 tablespoon shallots, diced

1 cup blueberries

2 tablespoons rice vinegar

1 tablespoon fresh grated ginger

Directions:

Preheat an indoor or outdoor grill over medium heat.

Brush the chicken lightly with olive oil and season with the onion powder and black pepper.

Place the chicken on the grill and cook approximately 7-10 minutes per side, depending on thickness, until the chicken is cooked through and no longer pink in the center.

While the chicken is grilling, add the remaining olive oil to a saucepan over medium heat.

Add in the shallot and sauté for 5 minutes. Next, add in the blueberries and cook, stirring frequently until the blueberries begin to break up.

Add in the vinegar and stir while the vinegar reduces for 2-3 minutes.

Stir in the ginger, and reduce the heat to low. Cook, stirring frequently for 3-5 minutes.

Remove the saucepan from the heat and brush the chicken once with the glaze while it is grilling.

Save the remaining glaze to serve with the chicken as an additional garnish.

Easy Bean Chili

Ingredients:

1 tablespoon olive oil

1 cup onions, diced

1 cup poblano pepper, diced

4 cloves garlic, crushed and minced

1 cup pinto beans, cooked or canned and drained

1 cup garbanzo beans, cooked or canned and drained

2 cups tomatoes, diced

1 teaspoon cumin

1 tablespoon chili pepper

1 tablespoon espresso powder

2 teaspoons dark cocoa powder

2 teaspoons paprika

1 cup low sodium tomato juice

2 cups low sodium chicken or vegetable stock

4 cups spinach, torn

Directions:

Heat the olive oil in a large stockpot over medium heat.

Add the onion, poblano pepper and garlic. Sauté for 5 minutes.

Next, add in the pinto beans, garbanzo beans and tomatoes.

Season with the cumin, chili pepper, espresso powder, dark cocoa and paprika. Cook while stirring for 2 minutes.

Add in the tomato juice and chicken stock. Mix well, and bring to a low boil.

Reduce the heat, cover and simmer for 10 minutes.

Add in the spinach and cook for an additional 5 minutes.

Broccoli Slaw

Ingredients:

4 cups broccoli

1 cup red onion

1 cup carrot, sliced

½ cup low fat plain yogurt

¼ cup Dijon mustard

2 tablespoon apple cider vinegar

1 teaspoon honey

1 cup edamame, cooked and shelled

½ cup almonds, sliced

½ cup pomegranate seeds

Directions:

In a food processor, combine the broccoli, red onion and carrot. Pulse until evenly shredded.

In a bowl combine the yogurt, Dijon mustard, apple cider vinegar and honey. Whisk until well blended.

Place the broccoli mixture in a bowl and add in the edamame, almonds and pomegranate seeds. Toss to mix.

Add the dressing to the bowl and toss until evenly coated.

Cover and refrigerate for at least 2 hours before serving.

Avocado Chocolate Popsicles

Ingredients:

2 avocados

1 ½ cup coconut milk

½ cup low fat vanilla yogurt

2 tablespoons honey

¼ cup dark chocolate, chopped

¼ cup pistachios, chopped

Directions:

Cut open the avocados, remove the pit and scoop out the pulp into a blender or food processor.

Add in the coconut milk, yogurt, honey, chocolate and pistachios. Blend until creamy. Transfer the mixture to popsicle molds.

Place in the freezer and freeze for at least 2-4 hours, or until firm, before serving.

Chocolate Pomegranate Smoothie

Ingredients:

2 cups low fat vanilla yogurt

½ cup brewed coffee

1 tablespoon dark cocoa powder

¼ cup pomegranate juice

½ banana

1-2 cups ice

Pistachios, finely ground for garnish (optional)

Directions:

In a blender, combine the yogurt, coffee, cocoa powder, pomegranate juice and ice.
Blend until creamy.

Transfer to chilled glasses for serving and garnish with ground pistachios, if desired.

Conclusion

The problem that we are experiencing with our current hypertension epidemic has many layers. We have to begin looking at the causes of high blood pressure and taking personal responsibility for the contributing factors that we can control. However, before we do that, we really need to look at high blood pressure and hypertension and serious conditions. Many people have a mindset that if your blood pressure is high, all you have to do is relax, change a few things and you will be fine. Even scarier is the fact that many people don't consider high blood pressure to be "that serious" of a condition at all. The truth is that high blood pressure can have absolutely devastating effects on your health and even the lives of your loved ones.

The intention of this book is to not only highlight the importance of recognizing and treating high blood pressure, but showing you an approach that is natural and instinctive. Treating high blood pressure can be as easy as adopting a new approach to eating that involves the superfoods listed in this book. The word superfood should not be confused with miracle cure, but it should be used to identify foods that nature has provided us with that work with your body to attain health, rather than against to destroy the very systems that keep you alive. Through this book, I hope that you feel invigorated, refreshed, informed and excited about taking control of your blood pressure concerns and regaining health, vitality and an incredible quality of life.

Made in the USA
Middletown, DE
08 January 2017